FERTILITY DIET RECIPES FOR WOMEN

A Comprehensive Guide With Delicious Meals To Boost Hormonal Balance And Empower Women Into Motherhood.

Jenny Pearl

Table Of Contents.

Introduction

In the delicate dance of life, the desire to embrace motherhood often intertwines with the importance of nurturing our bodies. "Fertility Diet Recipes for Women" is not just a cookbook; it's a guide to nourishing the foundation of fertility through wholesome and delectable recipes.

This book begins by demystifying the connection between nutrition and reproductive health. As we embark on the journey of fertility, understanding the role of key nutrients becomes paramount. The pages unfold with insights into the power of a fertility-friendly kitchen, emphasizing the impact of our culinary choices on the body's readiness for conception.

Breakfast becomes a vital chapter, unveiling recipes crafted to kickstart the day with energy and nourishment. From nutrient-rich lunchtime meals to savory dinner delights, each dish is carefully designed to support reproductive wellness. Snack smartly throughout the day with healthy bites that not only satisfy cravings but contribute to the overall fertility journey.

No journey is complete without a touch of sweetness, and this book introduces delectable desserts designed with fertility in mind. Beverages for balance take center stage, featuring infused drinks and teas to complement your fertility diet.

Meal planning becomes a breeze with practical tips and techniques, ensuring a seamless integration of fertility-boosting recipes into daily life. Delve into a chapter dedicated to exploring superfoods that go the extra mile in enhancing fertility. Tailored recipes for specific dietary preferences cater to diverse tastes and lifestyles.

Beyond the kitchen, the book delves into the importance of lifestyle habits that contribute to optimal fertility. Learn how to track progress, make adjustments to your diet, and embrace a holistic approach to nurturing your body for the exciting journey ahead. Frequently asked questions are addressed, offering clarity and guidance to those navigating the complexities of fertility.

In a world where every journey is unique, this book serves as a companion, providing not just recipes but a roadmap to empower your fertility journey. As you flip through the pages, discover the joy of creating meals that not only delight the palate but also contribute to the vitality needed for the incredible endeavor of bringing new life into the world. "Fertility Diet Recipes for Women" is more than a collection of recipes; it's a celebration of the intertwining threads of nutrition, health, and the timeless desire for the miracle of motherhood.

Chapter One

Understanding Fertility

Understanding fertility is like deciphering the intricate dance of nature within our bodies. It's a harmonious rhythm that involves a delicate interplay of hormones, reproductive organs, and overall health. In the context of "Fertility Diet Recipes for Women," grasping the basics of fertility sets the stage for a culinary journey that aligns with the natural rhythms of the reproductive system.

At its core, fertility revolves around the menstrual cycle – a monthly orchestration orchestrated by hormones like estrogen and progesterone. Tracking this cycle provides valuable insights into the fertile window, the optimal time for conception. The book introduces the reader to this cycle, demystifying the signals and rhythms that guide the journey towards parenthood.

Nutrition emerges as a key player in this fertility narrative. Essential nutrients, vitamins, and minerals act as the building blocks for reproductive health. From folate supporting fetal development to antioxidants protecting eggs and sperm, each nutrient plays a vital role. The book simplifies this nutritional puzzle, making it accessible for every reader, regardless of their familiarity with the world of nutrition.

Moreover, understanding fertility involves recognizing the impact of lifestyle factors. Stress, sleep, and physical activity all contribute to the intricate balance necessary for fertility. The book explores how simple lifestyle adjustments can positively influence reproductive health, complementing the power of nutrition in the fertility equation.

Through this exploration, the reader gains a unique perspective – fertility is not a distant concept but a tangible aspect of one's well-being. It's a holistic approach that embraces both the science and the art of conception. The simplicity lies in breaking down complex concepts into digestible information, empowering the reader to make informed choices on their fertility journey.

In the world of "Fertility Diet Recipes for Women," understanding fertility is not a prerequisite; it's an enlightening chapter that enhances the appreciation for the body's incredible capabilities. It sets the stage for a culinary adventure that aligns with the ebb and flow of fertility, making the journey towards conception both meaningful and delicious.

Chapter Two

Nutrient-Rich Foods For Hormonal Balance

In the tapestry of fertility, nutrient-rich foods play the role of vibrant threads, weaving a story of hormonal balance within a woman's body. "Fertility Diet Recipes for Women" unfolds a simple and unique narrative, highlighting the importance of these foods in nurturing the delicate dance of hormones.

Imagine a plate adorned with colorful vegetables, leafy greens, and fruits – this is where the journey towards hormonal equilibrium begins. Essential vitamins like Vitamin D, found in sunlight-kissed mushrooms, and Vitamin E from nuts and seeds, take center stage in supporting reproductive health.

Lean proteins, such as poultry and beans, provide a steady supply of amino acids, the building blocks for hormones. Whole grains like quinoa and oats bring a symphony of fiber, stabilizing blood sugar levels and promoting hormonal harmony.

Omega-3 fatty acids, found in fatty fish and flaxseeds, emerge as potent allies in the hormonal ballet, offering support for both fertility and overall well-being. The book's recipes artfully incorporate these nutrient-rich foods, creating a culinary masterpiece that not only delights the palate but also nurtures hormonal balance on the journey to conception.

In this exploration of fertility nutrition, simplicity meets uniqueness, and every bite becomes a step towards harmonizing the intricate hormonal symphony, creating an environment where the dream of motherhood can blossom.

Chapter Three

Power Of Superfoods In Boosting Fertility

Within the pages of "Fertility Diet Recipes for Women," the power of superfoods emerges as the unsung heroes in the quest for fertility. Picture them as nature's superheroes, each with a unique ability to enhance reproductive health in the simplest and most straightforward manner.

Blueberries, with their tiny yet mighty presence, are packed with antioxidants that combat oxidative stress, offering a protective shield for reproductive cells. Spinach, a leafy green champion, brings forth a rich source of folate – a superhero nutrient that supports healthy cell division and fetal development.

Quinoa steps onto the stage with its versatile prowess, delivering a punch of protein, fiber, and essential minerals. This superfood not only satisfies the taste buds but also provides a foundation for hormonal balance, a key player in the fertility journey.

Flaxseeds, akin to tiny magical seeds, bring a potent dose of omega-3 fatty acids. These little wonders contribute to the overall health of reproductive cells, creating an environment where conception can flourish.

In the simplicity of everyday ingredients, the book introduces the powerhouses like almonds, rich in Vitamin E, and salmon, a source of fertility-boosting omega-3s. These superfoods are not exotic or complicated; they are easily accessible allies in the pursuit of fertility.

The recipes within this book harness the inherent strength of these superfoods, blending them seamlessly into delicious creations. As readers savor the flavors, they also empower their fertility journey with the nutritional magic these superfoods possess.

In the world of fertility nutrition, simplicity reigns supreme, and the power of superfoods is revealed as a straightforward and unique path to enhancing reproductive well-being. Through the artful integration of these nutritional heroes, the book transforms meals into a celebration of fertility, making the journey towards conception both delicious and nourishing.

Chapter Four

Essential Vitamins And Minerals For Reproductive Health

Embarking on the journey of fertility, our bodies seek the guidance of essential vitamins and minerals as steadfast companions. "Fertility Diet Recipes for Women" unveils the simplicity and uniqueness of these nutritional allies, illuminating the path to reproductive health with clarity.

Vitamin D takes the spotlight, akin to the sun's gentle touch, fostering a fertile environment. Found in sunlight and foods like salmon and fortified dairy, it supports hormonal balance, a key player in the dance of conception.

Enter Vitamin E, the guardian of cell health, found in nuts and seeds. With its antioxidant prowess, it shields reproductive cells from oxidative stress, creating a resilient foundation for fertility.

Iron and folate join hands as a dynamic duo, present in leafy greens, beans, and fortified cereals. Iron ensures robust blood flow to reproductive organs, while folate offers a protective shield, crucial in the early stages of pregnancy.

Zinc, a quiet hero found in meat, seeds, and dairy, steps onto the stage, fortifying the immune system and aiding in the production of healthy eggs. Meanwhile, selenium, present in Brazil nuts and fish, supports the creation of DNA and shields against cell damage.

The simplicity lies in the everyday foods that house these essential nutrients, and the uniqueness is found in how effortlessly they become part of the fertility narrative. The book's recipes are a symphony of flavors, orchestrated to include these vital vitamins and minerals, transforming meals into a delicious investment in reproductive well-being.

In this exploration of fertility nutrition, the message is clear: the body's journey to conception is intricately linked with the nutrients it receives. The uniqueness lies in recognizing the profound impact of these essential vitamins and minerals in the simplest of foods, creating a harmonious melody that resonates with the dream of building a family.

Chapter Five

Hydration And Fertility Connect

In the fertility journey, hydration becomes a quiet yet crucial ally, weaving simplicity and uniqueness into the fabric of reproductive well-being. "Fertility Diet Recipes for Women" emphasizes the intimate connection between staying well-hydrated and nurturing the path to conception.

Water, like a gentle stream, plays a vital role in maintaining optimal bodily functions, including reproductive health. It aids in the transportation of essential nutrients, ensuring the body is a fertile ground for conception. Think of hydration as a sip of vitality, supporting the balance of hormones critical for fertility.

The uniqueness lies in the simplicity of incorporating hydration into the daily routine. The book encourages the joy of infused waters, where fruits and herbs add a burst of flavor while keeping hydration levels in check. It's a celebration of fluidity, where every sip becomes a small but meaningful step toward the dream of building a family.

As readers explore the pages, they discover that the bridge between hydration and fertility is one paved with clarity and ease. This book stands as a reminder that in the journey to conception, embracing the simplicity of staying well-hydrated becomes a source of nourishment for the body and a unique contribution to the tapestry of fertility.

Chapter Six

Meal Planning For Optimal Fertility

Meal planning becomes a compass on the fertility journey, guiding women towards optimal health and increased chances of conception in the book "Fertility Diet Recipes for Women." Simplicity and uniqueness intertwine as this guide unfolds the art of crafting meals that nourish both body and fertility aspirations.

The essence of meal planning lies in creating a harmonious balance of nutrients across the day. Each meal is like a brushstroke, contributing to the vibrant canvas of reproductive well-being. It's not about intricate charts and complex calculations; it's about embracing a simple rhythm that resonates with the body's natural cycles.

The book introduces the concept of fertility-friendly meals, where the combination of proteins, carbohydrates, and healthy fats dances in harmony. Breakfast becomes a powerhouse of energy, lunch a symphony of nutrients, and dinner a comforting melody that supports relaxation and rejuvenation.

Snacks take on a new role, offering a bridge between meals and maintaining steady energy levels. The simplicity of the plan lies in incorporating a variety of colorful fruits, vegetables, and whole grains, creating a palette that not only pleases the taste buds but also contributes to the intricate tapestry of reproductive health.

Uniqueness emerges in the adaptability of the meal plans to individual preferences and lifestyles. Whether one follows a vegetarian or omnivorous diet, the book provides a versatile approach that ensures the joy of eating aligns seamlessly with fertility goals.

As readers embark on the journey of meal planning, they discover that the key is not rigidity but rather a gentle flexibility that accommodates the ebb and flow of daily life. The book stands as a companion, offering a simple yet unique guide to meal planning that transforms each bite into a step towards the dream of motherhood.

Chapter Seven

Breakfast Boosters: Recipes For A Fertile Morning

In the enchanting world of "Fertility Diet Recipes for Women," mornings become a fertile canvas painted with simplicity and uniqueness. The book unveils a collection of morning recipes that embrace the dawn with a burst of vitality, weaving a tapestry of nourishment for reproductive well-being.

Start your day with a Sunrise Smoothie, blending vibrant berries rich in antioxidants, a banana for a potassium boost, and a splash of almond milk for added nutrients. This simple concoction becomes a delicious elixir, infusing your morning with fertility-friendly goodness.

The Fertile Oat Bowl takes center stage, combining hearty oats with a symphony of seeds – chia, flax, and sunflower – providing a dose of omega-3 fatty acids and fiber. Top it with a medley of fruits for a sweet touch that nourishes not just the body but also the dream of conception.

For those who savor a warm start, the Sunny Scramble beckons. Whisk together eggs, spinach, and tomatoes for a protein-packed breakfast that supports reproductive health. It's a savory delight, bringing the unique flavors of morning to your fertility journey.

The simplicity lies in the effortless preparation, ensuring that even the busiest mornings can be infused with fertility-boosting nutrition. These recipes are a testament to the idea that fostering reproductive well-being can be as delightful as the sunrise itself, setting the tone for a day filled with vitality and the promise of new beginnings.

Chapter Eight

Lunches That Love Your Body And Enhance Fertility.

Discover the joy of lunches that not only love your body but also dance in harmony with your fertility goals in "Fertility Diet Recipes for Women." These lunchtime delights are a celebration of simplicity and uniqueness, transforming meals into a nurturing embrace for reproductive well-being.

Dive into a Garden Goddess Salad, a vibrant bowl brimming with leafy greens, colorful vegetables, and a sprinkle of fertility-boosting seeds. This light yet nutrient-packed salad is a symphony of flavors that supports hormonal balance and cellular health.

Savor the Mediterranean Chickpea Bowl, a hearty and protein-rich creation that features chickpeas, olives, tomatoes, and a drizzle of olive oil. This lunch not only satisfies your taste buds but also contributes to a fertility-friendly feast.

The uniqueness lies in the simplicity of these recipes, where whole, fresh ingredients come together effortlessly. These lunches become a delightful ritual, a moment to nourish your body and honor your fertility journey. With each bite, you embark on a journey towards optimal reproductive health, turning lunchtime into a delicious affirmation of your dream to create life.

Chapter Nine

Dinner Delights For Reproductive Wellness.

Experience the joy of Dinner Delights in "Fertility Diet Recipes for Women," where simplicity and uniqueness converge to create meals that elevate reproductive wellness. These dinner recipes are crafted with ingredients that dance in harmony with the body's natural rhythms, turning evening meals into a celebration of fertility.

Indulge in the Bountiful Baked Salmon, a delectable dish rich in omega-3 fatty acids. This flavorful main course not only delights the palate but also supports hormonal balance, creating a nourishing foundation for reproductive health.

For a vegetarian option, savor the Quinoa Fiesta Bowl. Packed with protein-rich quinoa, colorful vegetables, and a zesty dressing, this vibrant bowl is a feast for both the senses and reproductive wellness.

The uniqueness lies in the simplicity of these dinner recipes, each designed to infuse your evening with flavors that contribute to fertility and overall well-being. With every bite, you embark on a culinary journey that aligns with the dream of creating life, turning dinner into a delightful ritual on the path to optimal reproductive health.

Chapter Ten

Snack Smart: Fertility Friendly Bites

In the world of fertility, every bite matters, and "Fertility Diet Recipes for Women" unveils a collection of simple yet uniquely crafted fertility-friendly bites. These small delights are designed to infuse your day with flavors that not only please the palate but also support the intricate dance of reproductive health.

Take a moment to savor the Crunchy Seed Mix – a delightful blend of pumpkin, sunflower, and chia seeds. These tiny powerhouses are rich in fertility-boosting nutrients, offering a unique crunch that satisfies snack cravings while nurturing your body on the journey to conception.

For a sweet indulgence with a fertility focus, try the Berry Nut Bliss Balls. Packed with antioxidant-rich berries, nuts, and a hint of sweetness, these bite-sized treats not only satisfy your sweet tooth but also contribute to hormonal balance and overall well-being.

The simplicity lies in the easy preparation, making these bites a convenient and delicious addition to your daily routine. The uniqueness is found in the thoughtful combination of ingredients, turning each bite into a small but meaningful step towards the dream of creating life. These fertility-friendly bites are a testament to the idea that even the smallest indulgences can play a big role in supporting reproductive health.

Chapter Eleven

Sweet Treats For A Healthy Fertility Diet.

Indulge in the sweetness of fertility with the "Fertility Diet Recipes for Women," where simple and uniquely crafted sweet treats become a delightful part of the journey towards conception. These desserts are more than just delicious; they are a celebration of reproductive health and well-being.

Savor the Berry Bliss Popsicles, a refreshing blend of mixed berries and yogurt frozen into a sweet and nutritious treat. These popsicles not only satisfy your sweet tooth but also provide a dose of antioxidants that contribute to reproductive wellness.

For a guilt-free pleasure, try the Cocoa Avocado Mousse. This velvety dessert combines the richness of avocados with the decadence of cocoa, creating a creamy delight that nourishes the body with healthy fats and fertility-friendly nutrients.

The simplicity of these sweet treats lies in their easy preparation, while the uniqueness is found in the mindful selection of ingredients. These desserts aren't just an indulgence; they are a flavorful affirmation of the fertility journey, turning every sweet moment into a small yet meaningful step towards the dream of building a family.

Chapter Twelve

Beverages That Support Fertility

Quench your thirst with fertility-boosting beverages as "Fertility Diet Recipes for Women" unfolds a chapter of simplicity and uniqueness in liquid form. These drinks not only hydrate but also contribute to reproductive wellness, making each sip a small celebration on the path to conception.

Start your morning with the Sunrise Citrus Elixir, a zesty blend of citrus fruits infused with a hint of mint. Packed with vitamin C and hydration, this refreshing elixir kickstarts the day while supporting immune health and hormonal balance.

As the day unfolds, indulge in the Berry Hibiscus Iced Tea, a vibrant concoction of berries and hibiscus petals. Rich in antioxidants, this iced tea not only cools but also provides a delicious dose of fertility-friendly nutrients.

For a soothing evening ritual, sip on the Golden Chai Latte. Turmeric, the golden hero, combines with warm spices and milk for a comforting beverage that carries anti-inflammatory properties and supports reproductive health.

The simplicity of these fertility-friendly beverages lies in their easy preparation, making them a delightful addition to your daily routine. The uniqueness is found in the thoughtful selection of ingredients, transforming drinks into more than just refreshment – they become a flavorful affirmation of the body's fertility journey.

Embrace the joy of hydration with these uniquely crafted beverages, turning every gulp into a small yet meaningful step towards the dream of creating life. In this liquid journey, simplicity becomes a source of nourishment, and each sip is a reminder that fertility support can be as easy as enjoying a delicious and thoughtfully crafted drink.

Chapter Thirteen

Weekly Meal Plans For Enhanced Fertility

Unlock the door to enhanced fertility with the simplicity and uniqueness of weekly meal plans in "Fertility Diet Recipes for Women." This guide transforms meal planning into a delightful and purposeful journey, crafting a palette of flavors that harmonize with reproductive well-being.

Begin your week with the Vibrant Monday Greens, featuring a kale and quinoa salad paired with grilled chicken. This meal plan kickstarts your week with a burst of nutrients and fertility-friendly ingredients.

Midweek, indulge in the Wholesome Wednesday Balance, offering a delightful mix of salmon, sweet potatoes, and steamed broccoli. This balanced combination not only satisfies your cravings but also nourishes your body with essential nutrients crucial for reproductive health.

Wrap up the week with the Relaxing Sunday Feast, featuring a comforting lentil stew and a colorful side of roasted vegetables. This Sunday meal plan is designed to provide a cozy and nutritious conclusion to your week, supporting relaxation and rejuvenation.

The simplicity of these weekly meal plans lies in their thoughtful curation, offering variety while focusing on fertility-friendly ingredients. The uniqueness is found in the adaptable nature of these plans, accommodating different tastes and preferences, making meal planning a joyous and personalized experience on your journey towards creating life.

Chapter Fourteen

Success Tips For Your Fertility Diet Journey

Embarking on your fertility diet journey in "Fertility Diet Recipes for Women" is a unique and empowering experience. Here are simple yet powerful success tips to guide you on this remarkable path:

- **Embrace Balance**: Let your fertility diet be a harmonious blend of proteins, carbohydrates, and healthy fats. Balance ensures a well-rounded intake of essential nutrients, creating an optimal environment for conception.

- **Colorful Variety**: Infuse your plate with a rainbow of colors. Different hues represent diverse nutrients, offering a spectrum of benefits for reproductive health. Aim for a vibrant and diverse array of fruits and vegetables.

- **Stay Hydrated**:Hydration is the unsung hero of fertility. Sip on water, herbal teas, and infused drinks throughout the day. A well-hydrated body supports healthy blood flow and hormonal balance.

- **Listen to Your Body**: Pay attention to hunger and fullness cues. Tune into your body's signals, allowing it to guide your eating patterns. This mindful approach fosters a positive relationship with food.

- **Include Superfoods**:Integrate superfoods into your meals. Berries, chia seeds, and leafy greens are nutritional powerhouses. These superfoods are like little guardians, supporting your body's fertility journey.

- **Plan Ahead:**Set yourself up for success by planning your meals ahead of time. Having a weekly meal plan simplifies grocery shopping and ensures you have fertility-friendly options readily available.

- **Celebrate Progress**: Recognize and celebrate small victories along the way. Every positive step, whether trying a new recipe or incorporating a fertility-boosting food, is a triumph on your journey.

- **Enjoy the Process**: Infuse joy into your fertility diet journey. Experiment with flavors, savor each bite, and view the experience as a celebration of your body's resilience and the anticipation of creating life.

By weaving these simple yet impactful tips into your fertility diet adventure, you not only nourish your body but also cultivate a mindset of positivity and joy on the path to realizing your dream of building a family.

Conclusion

Empowering women on the pathway to fertility.

In conclusion, empowering women on the pathway to fertility is not just about adopting a set of dietary recommendations; it's a journey of self-discovery and well-being. The essence of the "Fertility Diet Recipes for Women" extends beyond the kitchen, weaving together a tapestry of nutrition, mindfulness, and empowerment.

As we explored the diverse array of fertility-friendly recipes, we delved into the profound impact of wholesome nutrition on reproductive health. The simplicity of incorporating nutrient-rich foods like leafy greens, lean proteins, and whole grains echoed the notion that fertility is intricately connected to overall well-being. The book serves as a compass, guiding women to nourish their bodies in ways that support fertility naturally.

Beyond the culinary aspect, the empowerment lies in embracing the uniqueness of each woman's fertility journey. The inclusivity of the recipes recognizes that no two paths are the same, encouraging women to listen to their bodies and understand their individual needs. This personalized approach is the cornerstone of empowering women, steering them away from one-size-fits-all solutions and towards an understanding that their bodies are remarkable and unique.

Mindfulness emerges as a silent ally in the fertility journey, reminding women to cultivate a positive relationship with their bodies and minds. The simplicity of mindfulness practices integrated into the book fosters a sense of serenity amidst the sometimes challenging journey towards conception. Recognizing the emotional dimensions of fertility, the recipes become more than just nourishment; they become a vehicle for self-care and resilience.

In the realm of fertility, the power of community cannot be overstated. The book acts as a rallying point, fostering a community of women supporting one another. The shared experiences, tips, and encouragement create a tapestry of collective strength, dismantling the isolation that often accompanies fertility struggles. This sense of solidarity is a powerful force, propelling women forward with confidence and camaraderie.

The uniqueness of the "Fertility Diet Recipes for Women" lies not only in its culinary guidance but in its holistic approach to fertility empowerment. It reframes the narrative around fertility, shifting from a source of anxiety to a journey of self-empowerment. As women navigate the pathways of nutrition, mindfulness, and community support, they find themselves not only on the road to conception but on a transformative journey towards a more empowered and resilient self.

In its simplicity, the book invites women to embrace the power within, acknowledging that fertility is not a destination but a dynamic process. Through nourishing recipes, mindfulness practices, and a supportive community, women are equipped not only with tools for conception but with a holistic framework for lifelong well-being. The "Fertility Diet Recipes for Women" is more than a book; it is a companion on the empowering journey towards fertility, inviting women to discover the strength, resilience, and joy that reside within them.